GUIDE-TO-USE CIALIS

Understanding the Benefits, risks, and dosage management

DR. DANIEL ANDERSON

Table of Contents

CHAPTER ONE 3
    Overview of Cialis 3
    Ways to Take Cialis 18
CHAPTER TWO 27
    Errors to avoid 27
    Cialis Alternatives 31
    Preventing Possible Adverse Effects 43
THE END 51

CHAPTER ONE

Overview of Cialis

Cialis is one of the most often prescribed drugs for medical treatment of female sexual dysfunction and male erectile dysfunction. When patients attest to the goodness and efficacy of this drug, it is hardly surprising.

It works by increasing blood flow to all parts of the body, including the brain, spinal cord, and penis. This improved blood flow throughout the body aids in the prevention of a few systemic diseases, such as stroke and cardiac arrest. It even significantly reduces the risk of stroke along with various serious illnesses.

Cialis is thought to improve the brain's cognitive makeup, namely its capacity for understanding and absorption.

Cialis is a prescription that is given by a skilled doctor and comes in doses ranging from 10 mg to 25 mg. It is not a substance that can be used for self-treatment. The recommended starting dose for newbies is 10 mg, and the amount and duration of use will depend on how severe your erectile dysfunction is.

Cialis frequently loses its effectiveness, especially when taken with certain drugs. Most of the time, these combinations leave behind quite harmful side effects. As a result, people should never take Cialis along with any other drug without first seeking a licensed physician's advice.

Prominent Advantages of Cialis

The fact that the advantages of Cialis outweigh the risks is one important factor to take into account.

The main way that Cialis works is by increasing blood flow to the vaginal area and other parts of the body, which helps men get better erections and feel more satisfied during sexual activity.

In addition to its sexually stimulating effects, Cialis helps the heart's health and function. Constant circulation of blood along the central nervous system lowers the incidence of stroke and other spinal-related disorders.

In moderation, Cialis also reduces the risk of blood pressure.

Cialis enhances the sexual component of a relationship and the ambiance of that love relationship, allowing couples to practically realize their aspirations in a sexual setting.

Men's confidence can be increased, which is another advantage of using this medication.

It should be mentioned that Cialis doesn't make people sexually aroused; rather, it acts only once the individual using it is stimulated or becomes sexually aroused.

The benefits of Cialis start to take effect in less than 30 minutes, and the user is guaranteed a powerful, sustained erection for five hours.

Ways to Take Cialis

Once taken, Cialis takes around half an hour to start working, providing users about five hours of firm, sustained erections.

Make sure you discuss the advantages and disadvantages of using Cialis with a trained pharmacist or physician before beginning to use this potent drug.

In order to help you with your erectile dysfunction, your doctor might even suggest a dosage for you. Next, take your meds as directed by your physician or other healthcare provider. The best starting dosage for Cialis is 50 mg; this can go up to 100 mg based on the patient's tolerance level and the degree of severity of their sexual abnormalities.

Encouraging communication with your

physician and adhering to any prescribed follow-up regimen will go a long way toward eliminating any erectile dysfunction a patient may be experiencing.

It is recommended to take Cialis empty-handed, in contrast to other drugs. Steer clear of greasy foods when using this medication. The best time to take Cialis is when your body is consuming less fattening foods.

Overdosing on Cialis increases the chance of experiencing adverse effects like priapism, headaches, blurred vision, unconsciousness, etc.

Patients who abuse Cialis may potentially experience heart attacks and strokes. Use Cialis exactly as directed by your physician or pharmacist at all times.

Patients need to be aware of their surroundings and

report any negative consequences.

CHAPTER TWO

Errors to avoid

Do not cut short your doses simply because you are experiencing relief from erectile problems. Completing your doses helps to completely cure erectile dysfunction.

Avoid skipping your doses, or doubling them. Skipping those doses will slow down the effective pace of the medication, while doubling your doses drastically increases the amount of Cialis in your bloodstream.

Contacting a qualified doctor before starting the use of the medication is essential to fully understand the medication's uses, benefits, and how to dodge the risks through appropriate use of the medicine.

Cialis Alternatives

Men with erectile dysfunction can be treated with the prescription drug Levitra.

Like Cialis, it works best when taken on a vacant

stomach and comes in different sizes that vary from 5 mg to 20 mg.

After you experience sexual stimulation, Cialis takes around 40 minutes to become active and gives you a solid, long-lasting erection that lasts for about 4–5 hours.

There are a few minor adverse effects associated with using Levitra, including headaches, nausea, indigestion, and congestion in the nasal passages.

Refrain from taking Levitra with drugs prescribed for high blood pressure or chest discomfort in order to prevent negative interactions.

Cialis is another medication that is sufficiently potent to counteract the symptoms of erectile dysfunction.

It functions by boosting blood flow to the penis, treating erectile dysfunction, and strengthening men's erections. There are four dosages available: 2.5 mg, 5 mg, 10 mg, and 20 mg.

After taking Cialis for about 15 minutes, the user should expect a strong, sustained erection that lasts for 5–6 hours. Similar to Levitra, Cialis also has side effects that can be controlled by drug cessation or dose modifications.

To prevent negative interactions or associations, it's critical that you provide your doctor with a list containing all the medications you take.

Steer clear of taking Cialis along with high cholesterol and chest discomfort drugs.

Certain lifestyle changes such as regular physical exercises, and having a balanced meal can be adopted to cure erectile anomalies.

Mental issues like anxiety and depression can make it hard to achieve an erection. Engaging in therapy sessions could help tackle these mental issues.

Erections can be induced by injecting certain injections like alprostadil into the base of the penis.

Engaging in relaxation techniques or therapies like yoga and meditation can help relieve the mind of some mental and psychological issues.

Preventing Possible Adverse Effects

Since Cialis requires a prescription, it can't be used before first visiting a doctor.

The recommended dosages are given based on the severity of the erectile dysfunction in the patient. Follow your doctor's prescriptions exactly. Overuse causes adverse consequences including priapism, painful urination, extended erections, and excruciating migraines, among others.

Never take any medication with Cialis until first seeing your physician.

Never withhold any adverse effects from your physician; make sure to inform them of any reactions to the recommended dosages. If necessary, some modifications might need to be made to control the symptoms.

The effectiveness of the medications will be impacted if you skip or double the dosage; therefore, take them as directed by your doctor.

Even if your symptoms go away while taking the medication, make sure to finish all of your doses.

To speed up the healing of your erectile dysfunction, make sure you adhere to any additional physical and mental activity regimen or therapy prescribed by your physician.

THE END

www.ingramcontent.com/pod-product-compliance
Lightning Source LLC
Chambersburg PA
CBHW030055230526
45471CB00003B/1104